The F...NESS EXPERT Next Door

How to Set and Reach Realistic Fitness Goals in 10 Minutes a Day

By Michal Stawicki

www.expandbeyondyourself.com

September 2014
Copyright © 2014 Michal Stawicki
All rights reserved worldwide.
ISBN: 1508679932
ISBN-13: 978- 1508679936

Table of Contents

Introduction

I plan to make a series of booklets sharing my experiences of my life transformation. The one about weight loss is first. I am not a fitness guru; not even a personal trainer. I'm not a diet specialist. On the other hand, while not being any of the above, I did manage to lose 15 percent of my body weight (I'm a short and skinny guy; in absolute numbers, it is just 25 pounds). I can do 100 consecutive pushups, 54 consecutive dips, 33 consecutive chin-ups. And I didn't need any fitness guru, personal trainer, gym membership or diet consultant to do this. I didn't spend a lot of time or a lot of money. Weight-loss is just a by-product of my life's transition. And my fitness form is just a by-product of my weight loss.

I'm a busy person – a full-time employee (I spend about 18 hours a week commuting), father of three and a husband, a church community member, a blogger. But I discovered I don't need a lot of time (in daily terms) or money to lose weight. By sharing my story and advice, I want to convince you that you don't, either.

I intended this book to show purely my personal story, but then I ran across an old friend of mine that I hadn't seen in 10 years. He is also a busy father, husband and employee. And he lost about 12-percent bodyweight on his own. It made me think that my story is not so unique. Well, it is, of course, because every human being is unique; nonetheless, there are lots and lots of ordinary people's stories about getting fitter – people who changed their lives for the better.

I was already writing this book when I stumbled upon research published last year in the American Journal of Preventive Medicine showing exactly that. They surveyed over 4,000 obese people (BMI >29.9), among whom over 2,500 reported an attempt to lose weight. Over 1,500 got significant results. Research showed also that simple strategies were a greater success factor than participating in a commercial weight-loss program.

Over 60 percent of fatties who <u>attempted</u> to lose weight got significant results!

Weight-loss is not rocket science. It's not something reserved for the privileged, movie stars and TV presenters. Ordinary folks burdened with duties, jobs and families can do it, too. Thousands of people like you and me do it every year, every month, every day. Your neighbor did it. You can do it, too.

Les Brown said: "You will fail your way to success."

And he is so right! I failed my way to weight loss. I had vague thoughts about losing some weight as long as 5.5 years ago. I started seriously losing some pounds a year ago. 54 months of failure! I did everything backwards. I started from the totally wrong point and gradually drifted in the right direction. And I found tactics which bring results.

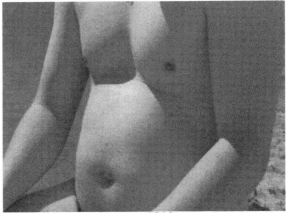
Summer 2011

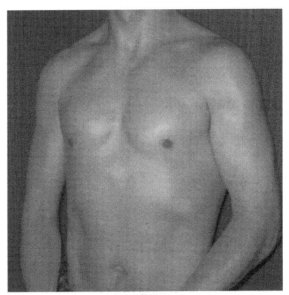
May 2013

I'm not going to impose my super-effective fitness program on you and charge $39 for it.

You don't need my knowledge to lose weight. Not that it is insufficient; it allowed me to get my results. The knowledge is at your fingertips – the Internet is full of diets, workouts and fitness programs. They work for some people; for other people, they don't. I don't accuse the fitness industry of preying on the naivety of their prospects. All those different programs have their advantages and are effective – under specific conditions. If you do what they say, when they say and in the way they say, you (usually) get the results. But the problem is, you must bend to those rules, and there is no universal detailed method which will work for everyone.

Imposing my rules on you will not be necessarily effective, anyway. For example, my wife decided to lose some weight when she noticed she was several pounds heavier than me. She asked me for advice. I answered, "Eat carrots as a snack," because that was what worked for me. She did it and got a stomach pain. I didn't even propose she follow the murderous workout program I practice, due to one simple reason – she hates physical exercises. From all the physical activities, the one she enjoys most is shopping. To be specific – shopping for outfits.

What you need is an incentive. An internal motivation. A story which will make you think that this is actually doable in your case, too. A few simple tips that will point you in the right direction. A fundament of "10 minutes philosophy," which you can make your very own life philosophy. This book is intended to help **you** to come up with **your** strategy – one that will work for you, so you can decide on your conditions, your time frames, your methods and your results. And above all, that will be believable for you, so you actually will start, will take action, based on this strategy.

10 Minutes

I'm deeply convinced that daily, consistent action absolutely must lead to results. Period. Well, to say that "I'm convinced" is putting it mildly. **I KNOW that daily, sustained action brings results.**

I know it because I do practice this rule in many areas of my life. I focus daily on specific actions, committing 10 minutes to them. I do track my results. And I do see them improving. I got results in such different areas as weight loss, finances, learning skills and relationships. I strongly suppose that it is a universal law applicable to absolutely ALL areas of life.

If you do something daily and you are not getting the desired results, it simply means you are putting at least as much daily and sustainable effort against those results. Let me give you a practical example. If you exercise 10 minutes a day, the same routine day by day by day, your muscles have to become stronger and your weight must drop, UNLESS, you counteract your exercises by introducing more calories to your diet, or by lying on the couch for the rest of the day.

The more action, the better results, up to some reasonable level - take a look at the chart below:

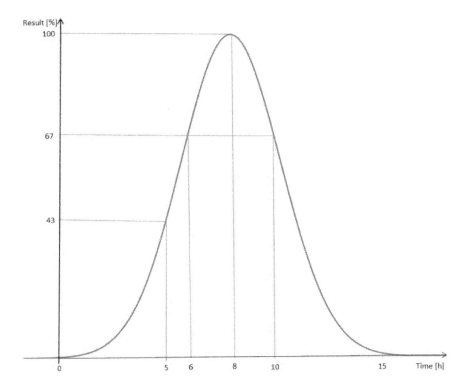

The shape of the curve is called normal distribution in probability research. It is in statistics something like the number π in math. As π can be found in many equations describing the texture of the universe, normal distribution can be used to describe a multitude of quantities in physics and measurements in biology, including IQ, height, weight and many more. According to central limit theorem, the mean of a large number of random variables tends to normal distribution. And in our big and complicated world, a lot of effects are presented by a large number of random data. I did study the statistics (years ago) and still don't understand most of this stuff, and it's out of the scope of this book, anyway. If you are curious, it is explained in a forthright way here: http://askville.amazon.com/Central-Limit-THeorem-apply-statistics-life/AnswerViewer.do?requestId=7620607

Firstly, to drive a point home (and to get away from scientific theories) please compare my pictures from the beginning of the book with the photos of my friend:

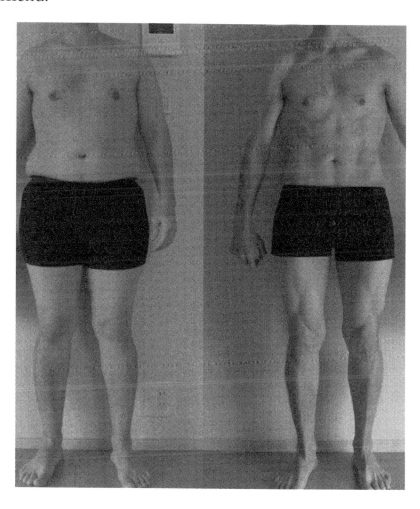

I lost about 25 lbs. in 10 months, Nathan lost over 40 lbs. within 90 days. I used about 25 minutes a day for my overall fitness program, his daily walk to a grocery store - and it was just a small part of his program - took him more than 30 minutes every day.

I believe the normal distribution can be also applied to describe a relation between a human effort represented by time and achieved results. We have to sleep, so we have about 16 hours at our disposal and we can get the maximum result investing half of them in one activity. If we give less time, we don't achieve the maximum result, and if we dedicate too much time, we are burning out.

But we are not going to devote 8 hours a day of our precious life to get the maximum result, which in this case would be ... a world bodybuilding championship, I suppose. We just need to shed some fat. Check out the zoomed left part of the first chart:

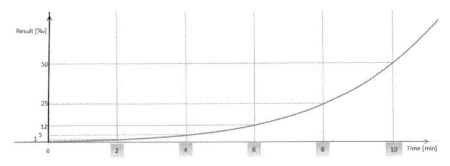

Even the smallest amount of invested time brings results. I consciously use about 2 minutes of my day on savings and I do a few monthly activities - a budget summary, paying bills, dividing my resources between different assets and so on - it takes me about 2 hours, so overall, it's 6 minutes a day. And it brings me the results. Quite recently, I met a guy who learned to play guitar practicing just 7 minutes a day. He has been doing it for three years and he is much better than me, although I have been playing a guitar for about 10 years. I just don't practice playing a guitar daily. My action is not sustained, so his results are more impressive.

Ten minutes is just a handy number. It can be two minutes and you still get the results. They'll just be microscopic and take around 50 times as long to see than if you had spent 10 minutes instead.

There are only two 100% effective methods to **not** achieve any goal: never start or give up (before you reach it).

But every - even the tiniest - consistent action brings result.

It's the core of this philosophy and it overcomes the two major obstacles of any lasting change: fear of failure, which stops us even before we begin, and giving up, which stops us after we begin, but before we get things done.

Every action brings results in the end. As long as you do something, you can't fail. There is no failure. You have nothing to fear. You can begin without the burden of hesitations and doubts.

And giving up is out of the question. What can cause you to resign, if you **know** that the results are inevitable, that all you need is just to sustain your action?

Giving up is not like an early withdrawal, where you get your money back, and sometimes even a part of the interest. It's like being in an investment program. Your obligation is to invest $1,000 every month, and if you do it for 5 years, you will get your $60,000 of capital and guaranteed $40,000 of the return on the investment. However, if you break the agreement you will get only part of your capital - from 10% in the first year of a contract to 50% in the last year - and none of the returns.

I'm fond of this simile, as it's not only about the process of getting results, but also, what you are going to do when you achieve them. After 5 years, you can decide on what to do with your money. You can put all of it back into the investment program again, or you can just spend everything. It's the same with any change in your life; it's the same with a weight loss. You can make yourself fit and then go back to your unhealthy habits and lose everything you've been doing for the last several months or years. Or you can build on it, for example by writing a Kindle booklet about a weight loss ;)

"All right" - you say - "but those are some fancy stories and theories. How is it applicable in my life?" I concur – theorization alone is quite useless. What caused me to embrace this philosophy wasn't other's stories and preaching. It was my own stories.

In order to feel at a gut level that it is indeed a universal law, applicable also to you, please give a thought to any successful area of your life. It can be anything - your marriage, a specific skill, a career, the fact that you have never had a car accident, good grades at school, a patience, your great relationship with your parents. The best thing for this little exercise is something you take for granted, but other people are praising you for. So, pick one and think: what makes you successful in this area? What's the difference between you and people who praise you, who aren't so successful? What do you do that they don't?

I bet you will find some consistent action underlying your success.

I take the love in my family for granted. I hadn't noticed it until my newfound online friends drew my attention to it by their comments on my personal blog. I have given it some thought and discovered that I say "I love you" to my wife and kids every day. When I was a teenager, I realized that, in my family, those words were ... well, maybe not a taboo, but close to it. I didn't hear those words very often at my home. And I was missing it. So I decided in my heart, that when I start **my** family, I will say this to **my** family members as often as I feel like it. It happened to be every day. In fact, several times each day. And this simple action makes all the difference in our family life.

And it's just one instance of this law. I have found many other examples behind my big and small successes - the high-school diploma, the scholarship on the 4th year of university studies, my personal fitness records.

It is true. You will find such examples in your life, too.

Look at the time/results chart once again. You probably noticed how the results grow exponentially after some point. As I said earlier - the more time you invest, the better results you get. I'm just assuming that weight-loss is not your first priority, so you don't want to invest much time. I understand you have your family to take care of, bills to pay, work to do, people to help, projects to attend to, relationships to keep or improve. A weight-loss comes after all of those activities in your life, so it's natural some additional pounds on your body have been developed. You have more pressing matters to take care of. You only have 24 hours and it's hard to find time for anything else. Thus, 10 minutes.

Philosophical Points to Remember

- every sustained action brings a result
- the keyword is "sustained," don't give up
- sustained action in the opposite direction will neutralize your good deeds
- find examples of the above truths in your life to embrace this philosophy on a personal level

Psychology

If you are a hardcore realist, feel free to skip this chapter. Just read the bullet points at the end. Remember however, that I've been there, done that. And I claim that your mindset is 80% of your weight loss.

Misconceptions about Weight Loss

I think there are a lot of false and sometimes even conflicting concepts about changing one's life, including, but not limited to:

- you need to have a monstrous will power
- you need a specific talent
- you need tremendous perseverance
- you need luck
    you need to work really hard to succeed
- you need to sacrifice a lot of time to get the results
- you need to get results fast or you will lose momentum and give up

– you need a big, challenging goal

And weight-loss is an area where all of these myths are really affecting people's minds. Don't get me wrong - all of the above points can be very handy in weight loss, but they are not critical. It's not that if you don't have luck or will power or a lot of time, then you can't lose weight.

A Reason to Change

What amazes me is that the key factor to any lasting change is so often overlooked: you need a compelling reason to change. I pinpointed a formula for any transformation:

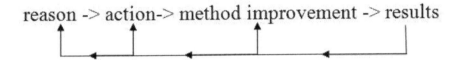

Each of the links in this "chain of change" is necessary. For example, without improving your method, you won't get good enough results to help you continue with your weight-loss program. Seeing that it doesn't work the way you wanted, you will just give up. Each one is also hooked up to the feedback loop.

Not a single component of this formula needs to be perfect, brilliant or impressive. It's enough that it leads to another step of the cycle. So **the only thing you need at the beginning is a reason, which will make you to take action**.

Everyone needs his or her own reason. My appearance wasn't a good enough motivator for me. I was getting rounder and rounder, but that didn't make me want to do anything about my weight. However, a little discomfort was enough to put me into action mode.

When I was 16 years old, I injured my spine jumping into a swimming pool. It was nothing serious, but when I got fatter, my strained spine began to hurt. The pain was annoying, coming back again and again in the least expected moments. And it was the reason I started my more than 5 year long quest for a weight loss. A friend of mine, who has already lost 37 lbs. and is on a quest to lose more, has a very similar reason: sedentary job, back pain. But my wife's reason was: "my husband can't weigh less than me!"

And I know you have your own, unique reason. If not, you wouldn't be reading this book.

The Snowball Effect

At the beginning, your expectations are not big, especially when you start with a firm decision to commit only 10 minutes a day. You just want to get rid of some fat from your body. So you start by developing a mundane habit like eating raw carrots as a snack. Then you start noticing changes and the snowball effect kicks in.

You can't even imagine what this small, insignificant discipline will bring to you. I just wanted to be thinner and pain-free. I got that and much more:

- I have a big Adam's apple. I felt strangled buttoning up my shirt collars. If I wanted to feel comfortable, I was forced to wear shirts one size bigger. But I lost fat from my neck and I can button up collars on all of my shirts. Neck fat! I would never have believed there was such a thing.

— my self-image skyrocketed. It's not that I had troubles with my self-image before. Why should I? I was just 8 lbs. above the 'normal' BMI boundary. I considered myself immune to such low opinions, the way I look does not determine my worth! I was wrong. I could be immune to the shallow judgments regarding obese people, but it came out that I'm not immune to those regarding muscular ones. I'm the same person inside, but I like myself more looking in the mirror and seeing a tough, muscular guy.

— my wife started her own weight-loss program, because "my husband cannot weight less than me" ;) And now she enjoys all the additional blessings of weight loss, too.

— I can run without much effort. I'm not a runner type. To give you the picture - my 10-year-old son is almost as fast as me (but he is the fastest among 10-year-old boys in his school). Yet, I need to jog quite often to catch a bus or a train, about twice a week. I used to feel exhausted; after each "race to the train," I was literally half-dead and out of breath. And now running feels terrific.

— the social acceptance of my transition is a great boost to my self-confidence. My friends and family are telling me they admire me, my efforts, my new look. As an adult human being, I shouldn't care much about other's opinions, but I do. Shame on me ;)

- I regularly beat my own fitness records - number of consecutive pull ups, pushups, dips. I like competing against myself. I like getting better results. I like my life more.
- my muscles showed up. I trained rigorously for years, but all my muscles were hidden under the layer of fat.

And that all is happening because I wanted to get rid of back pain. The reward is always bigger than you can imagine at the start.

You Are What You Think About

Embracing this simple truth will help you enormously in your weight loss. It's not just some hocus-pocus twaddle. Yes, I know you need to change your lifestyle, eating habits, introduce exercises. But those are secondary things. It's not 'going mystical.' It is about results.

I'm one of the most businesslike persons on this planet and that's why I'm putting a mind before a body. I know what I'm talking about - I got the best results not by a strict diet or an exhaustive training, but by applying a simple mental exercise which helped my mind to focus on the adequate physical means. I'm not saying that you'll lose your fat just by a hefty dose of daydreaming - absolutely not! The fat will not magically disappear, because you will cast a spell on it by the power of your mind. The physical means are necessary, they are just less effective alone or being put in the first place, before thinking.

I don't want you to become a master of your thoughts. Well, I do, but I'm not a master of **my** thoughts, so I'm not entitled to teach on that subject. I believe that conquering your mind and self-talk is a task much more intensive than losing some weight, and it's out of the scope of this booklet. You may be a god of a tiny part of the universe which consists solely of yourself. You can control it perfectly. However, this book is not intended to make you a Zen master, who controls himself absolutely, but to make you to start or enhance your weight-loss program. And to do it fast and relatively easy. I'm quite serious about "10 minutes" in the book's title.

I will not encourage you to say to yourself a hundred times a day: "I'm fit, healthy and fabulous," when you can clearly see your rolls of fat in the mirror. But you have to be conscious that your self-talk, this immaterial process taking part inside your head, **does** affect your outer world. Thinking: "I'm fat, I'm hopeless, I'm fat," a hundred times a day is not going to help you, either. Such thoughts are the shortest way to failure. How long, do you think, will you persevere in your commitment (even a 10-minute commitment) while being bombarded by those kinds of messages from the inside?

The right thinking **is** important. I've never doubted I can lose weight. Maybe it's because in my mind's eye, I had the skinny pictures of me from my adolescence. That's more or less what "The Secret's" gurus say.

Anyway, I had no doubts, so weight-loss seemed so easy to me. Persevering in my efforts for four years without visible results wasn't a problem for me.

Of course, you are a unique being and you can't borrow my mind set. It is just an example illustrating a victory of mind over matter. Looking from the outside, I was a hopeless failure. But my inner attitude got me through this experience to the point of getting some results. Don't dismiss the power of mind. Do not diminish it.

If you think in a wrong way, you won't even begin to take action.

Psychological Points to Remember

- you need a good enough reason for you to want to change
- your reason must ignite you to start an action
- you are not an animal; your thoughts **do** determine your actions
- your reason (and rewards) will grow with your weight loss progress

You Are What You Do

The thinking takes place before action, but it is action which brings results. You need right thinking or good enough thinking in the first place, so you'll take action, persevere and not give up. And that is 80% of success. The last 20% is proper action, skills and knowledge.

80% of action should be directed at the critical activities - more about that later. And it should be done in the right direction and steadily. As I explained before - you can't commit 10 minutes to your weight loss, then 30 minutes against it, and expect a positive net result. In other words - if you act that way, then what you do determines who you are. And you are not a weight loser anymore - you are a weight gainer.

Start Right Now

No amount of thinking will substitute for action. A few hours of thinking plus a few minutes of acting may do for the multitude. Months of thinking or dreaming without taking action is wasted time.

Going from the world of mind to the world of matter, from plan to action, is simple.

Just do it.

Take action.

Start today.

After each chapter, there are some bullet points. Pick one and practice it today.

Go and search for info. Do a set of pushups. Plan your diet. Schedule time for exercise. Buy different kinds of veggies to discover your tastes. Register on a weight-loss forum. Do something. Anything. Start gaining momentum.

There is no wrong way to start.

Persevere

Perseverance and consistency are necessary to achieve any results, at least in my world. I'm not talking here about quick fixes, winning the lottery, an extraordinary business proposal which will change your life without any initial investment and much work.

Get real. Be realistic. Get rid of marketing cataracts from your mind's eyes. Movie stars and politics don't really look as perfect as on TV. Heck! Most fitness gurus look at least a little worse in person than on their training videos. The Internet is full of 'get-rich-quick' schemes: "gimme your money and I'll show you how to get rich in no time!" Well, the disclaimers are there, too, of course. Put at the bottom of the page in fine print.

Our minds are bombarded by those kinds of messages all the time. And we are what we think about. We are all in a "get fit, rich, beautiful, happy and get it quickly" mindset. There are notable exceptions, but they are few and far between. Think of it. How many people do you know who exercise daily for at least one year? How many people who attend their church at least once a week for ten years or more? How many people who have a financial surplus? Compare those numbers to the number of people you know who visit Facebook every day, who watch TV every day, who eat sweets or chips every day.

We choose to satisfy our desires with quick and easy pleasures, instead of satisfying our needs by a sustained effort.

Behind 99% of success, there is certain to be hidden years of hard work, experience, blood, sweat and tears.

I know a story of a dentist who became a very successful Internet marketer. He sells the blueprint for other dentists on how to establish a profitable dental assistant school. Within 14 months, he sold this blueprint to over 50 locations. There were just 300 names on his list when he made his first launch and he made $140,000. The second launch to the list of almost 700 brought him another $90,000. Can you imagine what a clever marketer could do with such a story? I can see those imaginary headlines: "Make over $128 to $450 per your list member!" "Financial success in 14 months!"

And a fine print disclaimer at the bottom of the page: "We cannot guarantee anything, but you can achieve best results if you are a dentist (at least seven years of study!), start your own practice, start a dental assistant school working your butt off in the evenings after your practice for several years and then structure, systematize, market and sell a blueprint for such a school program."

Doesn't sound so inviting anymore, huh? But a dentist I'm talking about did exactly that. He worked 12 years to get to a point where he monetized his hard work. His first attempt to sell a blueprint through the Internet was unsuccessful - he sold just two products within a year. How would he be if he gave up the idea then? Well, $230,000 worse off.

You and I both know that this is the way to get the things done in the real world. Begin, work continuously, work hard, work smart, work as long as it takes to get the results. And there is no "give up" in this formula.

No matter if you invest 10 minutes a day or 10 years of your life into some venture - giving up will have exactly the same effect - null, nada, zero, zilch.

As long as you continue your commitment, there is a chance to succeed. The moment you stop is the moment this chance is lost. Never give up.

There are several reasons we usually give up, and the 10-minute philosophy can help you to beat up all of them.

- we give up because the task seems to be big and scary, just too hard to do. Well, in this instance, it's just 10 minutes, how hard could it be?
- we give up because it looks like achieving the result will just take forever (well, it's only several weeks or months, but we live in the Internet,

impatient era, we want it <u>yesterday</u>). But it will not take forever. It will take 10 minutes and your result (for today) will be achieved.

— we give up because our motivation drained. And it's much, much easier to motivate yourself for a 10-minute task than it is to lose 15% of your bodyweight in the next 10 months.

All in all, perseverance connotes with a long, hard, monumental job to do, and a mere 10 minutes is no such thing, is it? It's trivial.

OK, a photo to illustrate the point (one picture is worth more than a thousand words):

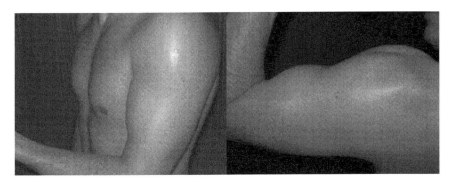

Those muscles were built by the thousands and thousands and thousands of pushups. I had been doing them when I was a fatty. They weren't done in one moment, day, week, month or even a whole year. It was several years. What is more, until quite recently, I did just one single consecutive series of pushups a day, which took me just 2-8 minutes. I would never have seen those muscles if I had given up doing pushups before losing my layer of fat.

Be Creative

We've covered the critical parts of taking action - firstly start, then never give up. However, which action you take is also pivotal. Don't get yourself locked into a certain kind of acting, which doesn't bring you results. It's not enough to be positive in your thinking and to take continuous action. Those elements are necessary, but if your actions drive you in the wrong direction, no amount of activity will achieve your weight-loss goal.

Let's compare weight loss to a voyage. It's not enough to define the destination, start the engine and move forward - you must drive in the right direction to reach your goal. If you took a wrong turn, being persistent will do you no good. You must make a U-turn, drive back and correct your route.

Be flexible with your approach.

You know best what's good for you. You know your circumstances, attitudes and fancies. And you are the best person in the world to compose your weight-loss program. If you like physical exercises, you can find an appropriate training on the market and use it, not the other way around: to buy a training and then make yourself do it against your predispositions.

It might happen, that once you commit to your weight-loss activities and do them for an extended period of time, you will find that you enjoy them or enjoy the results to such an extent that you are actually willing to put more of your resources into your program, more time or more money. But that's for the future. I was willing to give more only after three years. But being 'cheap' about my program did wonders for my creativity. I give you some examples to enhance yours:

1. I'm a fan of short, intensive exercises. I mean really short and really intensive. Usually, I do a consecutive series of one routine to the point I can't do even one more repetition.

I started doing pushups regularly 5.5 years ago. For the first two years, this simple exercise was enough for me. I did one consecutive series - as many pushups as I could. I started from about 40 and reached about 130. But man (oops! sorry gals), that took time! And I don't mean, it took me 2 or 3 years to reach 130 consecutive pushups level, but it took me about 7-8 minutes to finish the exercise. So I started to introduce changes to my routine - first, it was narrow-grip pushups, then diamond pushups, then all of the above with legs elevated. All of them were harder to do than normal pushups, so the time of my 'training window' stopped growing and even shrank a little.

I was doing over 80 legs-elevated pushups when I got the idea to put my kids on my back. Jackpot! My trainings started to be shorter and more intensive at the same time.

Unfortunately, I wake up for the morning shift about 5 a.m., and my children are not available so early. What is more, my wife complained that my exercises are too loud, my gasping for air wakes her up. Instead of giving up my work outs, I came up with a different idea. Being on the morning shift, I started to do dips instead of pushups. At the beginning, I was able to do about 20 consecutive dips. Again, it was faster and I made less noise. I used (and still use) my kitchen chairs as bars.

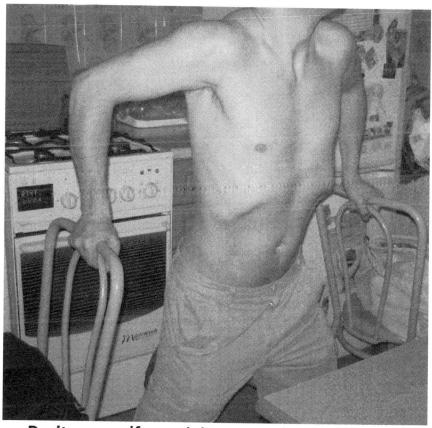

Do-it-yourself creativity example: chairs dips

2. About 2 to 2.5 years ago, I bought a bar for pull ups, the cheapest stuff from the supermarket (less than $10). And it stayed hidden behind the bed for six months, because I had no drill to install it with. At last, my mate, who is a carpenter, installed it when he was fixing some furniture in my apartment. Pull-ups are just great, they are the shortest workout I can imagine doing using only my body weight. At the beginning, I did just 14 chin-ups.

3. When I came to a doctor with my spine problem, she advised me to work on my belly muscles. I got fired up with excitement dreaming about sexy abs. But what to do? Sit-ups? I did 100 and felt I could do more! It appeared that pushups are great for belly muscles, too. So I found another body weight exercise -Weider series - and started to use it. Right, my belly muscles were strained, but soon the exercise took more and more of my time. And I didn't have the time. So I created it. I set an alarm clock 15 minutes earlier. I had already been waking up terribly early - about 5 a.m. - and 15 minutes made little difference. Unfortunately, I discovered that having sexy abs is hard to accomplish with just a quarter of a body-weight exercise.

4. I'm the one with a sweet tooth. Maybe even THE one. I could easily eat two pounds of cake in one afternoon. I love sweets. I'm an addict. When I realized I need to change my diet, it was quite easy to target my vice. But what to do with that? I've come up with an idea to at least partially replace sweets with raw carrots. Why carrots? They are cheap, available all year long and I like them. Whenever I had an urge to eat something full of sugar, I took a carrot instead. That was the first trigger allowing me to shed several pounds.

5. Then, I realized I don't know much about healthy eating and diets. Up to that point, it was "a woman's thing" for me. I did some research on the Internet.

Under the layer of mystical spells I found the bottom line - calorie intake. I found a great website where I can check almost every scrap of food for the number of calories. I paid attention to what I eat. I composed a reasonable daily diet from the foods I eat and like. I reduced the amount of bread I ate by about 25%. You might ask: what's so creative about that? Well, I made my own plan of meals. I didn't choose any specific diet, imposed from the outside. And because it was mine, I stuck to it.

6. You need to be committed over a long period of time to get results, especially if your energy or effort input is low.

I was still looking for any additional methods or tools I could use, as I still wasn't satisfied with the output.

I don't remember where I got the idea of a food journal, or as I call it - a diet log. For sure it was not mine. Anyway, I started to keep it on the 3rd of January 2013. It's a very simple tactic and from the rational perspective, it shouldn't make any difference at all. I didn't burn many calories writing on a computer's keyboard for three minutes a day, I didn't change my workout regime or diet. However, it made all the difference. I've achieved my dream weight two months and six days later.

Action Points to Remember

- start right now!
- persevere
- monitor your methods and progress; adjust them, if necessary
- be creative

Two "Dark Secrets"

There are just two very secret rules of weight loss hidden in safe deposits of fitness gurus, so we common mortals cannot reach them and be fit. I will reveal them right now and revolutionize your life forever. Those rules are:

— eat less

— move more

The more important one is "eat less." If you are not anorexic or bulimic, bending to this rule will give you the best results.

Eat less

If you take just one piece of data from this book, this one is the most important in weight loss: **Proper eating is 80% of your weight-loss success.** Your eating habits, your foods intake, determines the output of your fat-loss efforts. "Eat less" is a magic formula for losing weight, if you look for one. There is no other.

The prevailing strategy (65% responses) among respondents of the research I mentioned at the beginning of this book was: eat less. The research showed also that it was more efficient than participating in a commercial weight-loss program.

Weight-loss can be reduced to a simple math formula – it is all about the number of calories you eat and burn. There is more to it of course - your body assimilates different types of food at a different pace, your digestive system works more efficiently at specific times of day, physical exercises can boost your metabolism, and so on. However, the bottom line is to maintain the calorie-deficit, and it can be represented by a formula:

calories eaten - calories burned = weight loss

But what really makes this formula less practical is an unpredictable human behavior. For example, the advice not to eat late in the evening has to do less with our metabolism and more with our attitudes. Yes, your body works slower while you sleep, but it doesn't mean your supper will be mysteriously transformed into fat tissue. Your body just needs more time to digest it. What is really dangerous in late eating is the types of food we usually consume then: junk food, snacks, sweets, alcohol. Thus, the weight-loss researchers could easily connote night-eating with obesity, and conclude the finding that one leads to the other.

I've told you before about my friend who lost 37 lbs. I asked him: "What method have you used?" He answered: "The scientific method. I ate less calories than my body used." And because he believed that, he could dismiss all the contradicting philosophies - eat this, don't eat that; eat six small meals, no, eat just two and apply intermittent fasting; eat fruits on an empty stomach, no, use them as snacks - and focus on the bottom line, which is calorie intake. I'm not saying some of them are not valid or at least valid in specific circumstances, but they are just minor details in your weight loss. It doesn't matter what you eat or when you eat, if you eat too much!

So, use the "scientific method" of my friend. Focus on how much you eat, know your daily calorie intake. That's your grand strategy. Types of meals, time of meals and their frequency are mere tactical means.

I can easily read your mind right now: "But what do you mean eat less? Are you advising me to starve? I eat just enough to function normally, I'm not overeating!"

Well, you **think** you are not overeating. Exactly as I thought before my weight loss quest. I'll tell you this: If your BMI result is above 26, then you **are** overeating. Take a look at my fat photo at the beginning of the book. The man you see there is not obese. I was just a little overweight - just several pounds. And I **was** overeating. So if you are anything like me from the photo, or bigger, there is still leeway. Thoughts of starvation is just a whining of your subconscious mind, which is trying to protect you against any changes. The primal fear of hunger is rooted deep inside us, but let's face it - it's not the hunger which is a safety hazard to our life today, it's an overconsumption.

Five years ago, I used to eat four double sandwiches of white bread at work:

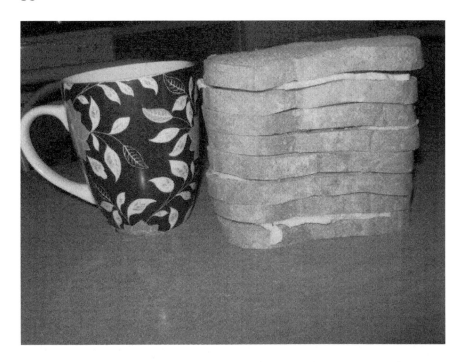

I also ate a breakfast and a late lunch at home. And a doughnut about every 2-3 days. And a cake every time there was an occasion to eat one. And some sweets in the evenings. Compare the amount of food I then ate with my today's diet:

- 3 slices of whole grain bread with ham. A big cup of tea with one spoon of sugar and rum
- 2 chops of chuck with potatoes and onion
- 4 chips
- 2 jellybeans
- one orange
- one carrot
- 4 slices of whole grain bread with honey. A big cup of chicory coffee with milk

So, I ate less and I survived. Well, I thrive, in fact. I have never felt better physically in my life. I can comfortably wear my wedding suit (I've been married for almost 13 years). I'm beating my fitness records like crazy - about a dozen since January; four while writing this booklet. I've beaten the last one on the 2nd of July - 29 consecutive pull-ups. I'm in better shape than I was 15 years ago.

You can eat less. It's possible. You must eat less in order to lose weight. If you still have a problem with that thought, if you still feel restricted, let me tell you a story which will put some light on this subject.

Some time ago, I think it was November 2012, I watched a TV program about obese people losing weight (my wife enjoys watching such shows on "the woman's" channel). Most of them did that by stomach stapling. But there was one guy who lost 400 pounds without any surgery or pharmacology. He told his philosophy of weight loss: "Eating is my addiction. I think it is the worst addiction of all, as eating itself is necessary to support my body with energy. I cannot break up with it, like with drugs or alcohol." He overcame his urges in the simplest possible way - he has only the food for his nearest meal at home. After a breakfast, he goes to the grocery to buy his lunch. After a lunch, he goes there again to buy his supper.

By the way, this is the same tactic Nathan (my friend from pictures in chapter 2) used to achieve rapid results in his weight-loss. He goes to the grocery every day to buy the food products only for the next day, too.

I sympathize with the TV show guy's philosophy. That kind of attitude to eating, especially to consuming sweets helped me enormously in my weight-loss. I'm a lifelong, irredeemable, sweets addict. I needed to recognize that truth to take measures against it. You, too, need to recognize the truth about your bad eating habits before fixing them.

Please do understand the moral of the story properly. Overly stressing out about what, how and how much you eat can be disastrous to your health, too. We all know the stories of anorexic or bulimic media celebrities, don't we? Jim Rohn in "Cultivating an Unshakeable Character" instanced a long-term Finnish research comparing the health of two groups of people. Members of the first group could eat what they wanted. The second group was closely supervised – they could eat only healthy foods and in specific quantities. The stress related to tracking and controlling their eating caused more damage to their health than a "free" diet to the health of the first group's members.

Every extremity is dangerous. But most of our society, me two years ago and probably you reading this book, are just on the other side of extreme. We are absolutely careless about what and how much we eat. We don't think about it at all. To the effect, we eat too much. And that's the reason for our fat rolls.

Eating less is not a whim, it's the absolute bottom line of weight loss. **If you still feel rebellious about it, your first task is to overcome this feeling.** You will waste your time and energy attempting to lose weight with such an attitude. Don't buy a gym membership, don't look for magic pills or diets, don't start regular workouts - it all will be in vain, if you won't eat less.

Go and find your philosophy, the kind of thinking which will make you accept that eating less is not depriving you of life's pleasures, but giving you the lifestyle you want. The new, healthy and fit you. Find your deep reason. As I said in Chapter 3, it doesn't have to be big, just big enough to change your attitude and ignite you to start taking action. For my wife, the motivation is her conviction, that her husband shouldn't weigh less than her. Sensible? Not necessarily. "Good enough" to start an action? In her case: yes.

So, eat-less rebel (if you are one) - if you want to lose weight, the best way to start is investing your 10 minutes in the search for your philosophy. Keep looking until you find something stimulating you toward eating less. You don't have to become a fanatic of fasting. You just need to be comfortable with the fact that consuming less food is actually serving your purposes.

OK, enough is enough. We talked about "10 minute philosophy," about mind set, about the upmost importance of eating less in weight loss. Now, it's time to show you a technique which will both take you less than 10 minutes of your time, and bring big results. I did everything backwards and I want you to get much better results by doing things in the proper order. This is the first and foremost tool you should use. It is efficient even when you use it as a last resort, as I did, but why wait? Start out with it and you will see the change on the scale much faster than me.

Keep a Diet Log

An incentive may be the first thing, but actual diet regime is important, too. If you didn't pay attention to your eating habits at all, you might have no idea as to what to cut out from your menu.

So it's time to introduce you to a diet log.

It's nothing innovative. It's known under many names: a food journal, a diet diary - just to name a couple. You use this simple technique by writing down everything that you eat and drink which contains calories. Every scrap of bread, every cookie, every glass of soda - everything. It is simple. It is mundane. It works.

Take it seriously. Make a plan how to go about it. Analyze your day, your eating patterns and decide on your tactic. You don't need an elaborate scheme or refined technical means. Keep it simple. Use a pen and a pocket notepad, iPad, a mobile phone - whatever suits you. It must be something you feel comfortable with and is easily accessible most of the time.

I spend more than a half of my life in front of a computer, so I found it congruent to log my food intake in a text file. If I was without computer access, I jotted down what I put into my mouth on a piece of paper, and later on typed it into a diet log file.

Take a look at a weekly excerpt from my log: http://www.onedollartips.com/dietlog/ That week, I lost a little more than one pound.

There are diet logs and diet logs. Some people write down a time of meal, the exact number of calories and how much water they've had. I just jotted down the amount and type of food and drink. I found it a "good enough" solution, as I wasn't supervising the Olympic Master fitness program, but an ordinary (and busy) man's weight-loss program. The main reason for keeping a diet log is to be aware of what and how much you eat. Being mindful makes miraculous changes to your behavior. Calculating the exact number of calories you consumed may be an additional feature, but one you need to put additional effort (and time) for.

Do treat keeping a diet log as a test of your real intentions. If you don't do it, you don't really want to lose weight; you are just playing with a thought to do it.

I mean, here I am - an expert. At least from your point of view, I'm assuming you are a reader who wants to lose weight – and I've already done it. I've managed to shave off fat, build some muscles and I've stuck with those changes. What is more, I did it with only marginal external guidance and by investing a minimal amount of time and resources. I made many mistakes along the way and I want you to avoid them, to choose the optimal path. And I'm telling you to do the simplest thing anyone is capable of doing. I insist it is important.

So, if you are not going to do it, what is that saying about your attitude? Are you really serious about your commitment?

You may come up with some reservations about a diet log, but you know what they really are? Excuses.

Get serious. Get the job done. I'll help you by shooting down some excuses:

- I don't have time.

OK, I know. That's why I asked you to keep a diet log. It's the fastest, easiest and most efficient method to lose weight. You must be crippled or eat every 30 minutes to spend more than 10 minutes daily on your diet log.

- It's a lot of trouble.

Really? How? Carrying a pen and notepad is trouble for you?

- It is stupid hocus-pocus. No one lost even an ounce of fat by writing down things on paper!

I did. What is more, a food journal is a part of many, many commercial fat-loss programs. Are you suggesting they are kidding their clients?
And you don't have to track every crumb going into your mouth for the rest of your life. It's a tool to make you aware of your eating habits. I've been keeping my diet log for about 85 days. I quit it two weeks after achieving my dream weight. But my mindfulness is at a high level to this day. I can recall everything I've eaten in the last 24 hours. So keep it as long as you need to develop your mindfulness.

Eat Less Points to Remember

- eating is 80% of success in weight loss

- calorie intake is a grand strategy
- you over-eat
- eating less will fit you, won't kill you - adjust your mindset accordingly
- keep a diet log
- treat a diet log as an indicator of your commitment to lose weight

Move More

According to the 80/20 rule, to move more is the less critical factor in weight-loss, responsible for only 20% of your results. That's good news for anyone who hates to exercise. It's quite possible and achievable to lose weight without any additional physical activities.

However, as you have to eat, you also have to move. It's impossible to live without those functions. Why don't you use it to your advantage? Each additional pound of muscle will burn an extra 45-50 calories a day. So I encourage you to go and gain those few additional pounds of muscle. The beauty of it is that you need no additional equipment or time to do it. All you need is a mindset which constantly looks for opportunities to move more in your everyday activities, a consciousness about your lifestyle.

Are you going to play with your children? Go and play basketball, instead of a board game.

Are you going to the mall? Park at the farthest parking spot, instead of close to the door.

Are you going to the 3rd floor? Take the stairs, instead of an elevator.

With an "active mindset" you will find plenty of opportunities to move more. Remember the weight-loss formula:

calories eaten - calories burned = weight loss

Every single additional physical activity brings more burned calories to this equation.

I encourage you to start to work out daily. Bodybuilders insist on exercising every few days, so the muscles can rest and recover. But we are talking here about a few minutes workout, not a bodybuilding. Daily exercise will develop into a habit in half the time, compared to doing it every other day. You can go softly and gently like my wife, who hates moving. Do some aerobic routines for a few minutes every day. Or, you can go hardcore like me - choose an exercise and do a consecutive series to max out.

HIIT

As I mentioned before, I'm a fan of short and intensive trainings. I figured it out wholly on my own - I was so proud of myself - only to find out that I'm not a fitness genius. There are others who cleared the path long before me. It just shows how detached from anything resembling a healthy lifestyle I was. So, what the heck is HIIT (High-intensity interval training)? According to the definition, it's "an enhanced form of interval training, an exercise strategy alternating periods of short intense anaerobic exercise with less-intense recovery periods," But try to ask how to do it, and you will get almost as many answers as there are people. I've literally seen people arguing on fitness forums:

"That's how you are supposed to do it."

"No man! It's done this way!"

"Guys, what are you talking about? It's not HIIT! Here is the link, where my guru is showing how to do it properly!"

Well, you get the picture. My mentor, Craig Ballantyne, has in his offer a Home Workout Revolution program including a four-minute workout called by a fancy name: "Max Rep Miracle Bodyweight." And, as far as I know, it is the only four-minute workout in his program. Four minutes? For me, it's almost too long.

Try to put a 115-lb. boy on your back, and do pushups for four minutes. Good luck. Or grab a bar and do chin ups for four minutes. Possible, some guys can do just that, but they are not ordinary mortals burdened by 9 to 5 jobs.

The bottom line of HIIT is: it's short, it's intensive. It makes your heart pound; it makes you gasp for air.

So, my very own and original ® way to do a workout is: one consecutive set of bodyweight exercise to your limit. And beyond. It's a little similar to Tabata workout, especially in the case of pushups. I do as much as I can, then I catch my breath on straight arms, and do some more. Straight arms, catch my breath and some more pushups. I do it until I'm breathless and powerless and I can't straighten my arms, I can't heft my body from the floor. It's doable with dips, too, but not in the case of pull ups. That's why I love them – this is the only exercise where my muscles give up before my lungs do.

I'm no fitness trainer, but the results I'm getting aren't too bad. Exercising only by this method, I've beaten Craig Ballantyne in pull-ups. He set a challenge in the Transformation Contest to do the maximum number of pull-ups within 8 minutes. I've beaten him by 6 pull-ups. I prepared myself better for this exercise, and a few days later, I beat him by 19 pull-ups.

I was blown away! He is a professional fitness instructor – it's his business; it's his life. Me? I have a bar in my apartment and at that time I practiced pull-ups 4-5 times a week, one series of consecutive pull-ups. That's all.

I'm a living example that a very short and intensive workout is at least as effective as long and low-intensive are. So why waste my (and your) valuable time on them?

Since I'm thin and fit, I feel better about myself, so I've actually expanded my workouts. I do my morning HIIT workout as usual, then 2-4 more workouts during the day, and a consecutive series of pull-ups. The reason for this additional exercise is my sweet tooth; thanks to all of those workouts, I am able to burn down a chocolate bar or two.

I recommend a HIIT workout to you. If you value your time, don't spend it on jogging or walking. Well, of course, do spend it on those activities if you enjoy them and you have time for them. But if you look for biggest gains in the least possible time, HIIT is definitely something you should consider.

I do my HIIT workout early in the morning. It has several advantages:

- it is relatively easy to find several minutes for an exercise; you just wake up a few minutes earlier
- you work out on an empty stomach; with high intensity training, it's a blessing. I can never max out, if I have eaten before
- it's easier to structure your morning and develop a habit than to do it later in a day, when your family, friends and job are fighting for your time
- it boosts your metabolism for the few first hours of a day

Move More Points to Remember

- an additional pound of muscle will burn 45-50 calories a day
- use your everyday activities as opportunities to move more
- exercise daily
- exercise in the morning
- for the fastest results, go for HIIT, if you dare

Practical Tips

1. If you never-ever tried to lose weight, try to start purely from your consciousness and mindset. Ask yourself the questions below every evening before going to bed. It will count as your 'only 10 minutes' given to a weight loss program:

- do I exercise every day? every 2 days? a few times a week? once a week? less than that?
- do I know how many calories I've eaten today?
- did I eat fast food today? any sweets? (if possible, numerate them all)
- did I eat vegetables/fruits today? how many? (if possible, numerate them all)
- how much water do I drink every day? how much today?
- how many hours did I sleep today? what is my average?
- what do I say to myself about my diet? my exercise routine?

If you answered for any self-check question: "I don't know," that's a very honest answer. And it immediately leads to another question, which can create your short-term action plan: How can I become aware of it?

Do this for 30 days in a row and check how this internal, mental activity affects your real world.

2. Weigh yourself regularly and in similar circumstances. I weigh myself every Saturday morning, before breakfast and after my morning workout. My cheap, piece-of- supermarket-art scale shows different weights in different locations. It shows 3 different measures, even in the same room. So I do my weighing in a bathroom, where there are stable floor tiles. I weigh myself 3 times and take the average. All this fuss is necessary to get objective information.

If you use different scales, at different places and times of the day, the feedback information you get is almost useless. The same place, the same time, the same circumstances guarantee obtaining quality information.

3. Use an online service to educate yourself about foods' nourishment and calories. Almost every weight-loss platform offers a foods library with pictures and such data. Sparkpeople.com, Livestrong.com - to name just a couple. I recommend http://caloriecount.about.com - the photos may not be 100% what the text describes at the moment, which can be misleading, but the access is totally free - no registration required.

4. Get literate in weight loss & fitness terminology: calories, BMI, carbs, HIIT, Tabata, cardio.

5. Move more on a daily basis. Do small, simple things daily: take stairs instead of an elevator; walk to the shop instead of driving; park your car further; put something heavy (like a big bottle of water) into your bag - you will carry additional weight with you - and so on. Done one time, it doesn't make much of a difference. Done every day, it really compounds over time.

6. Ask for advice. I made my own program, learning from my own mistakes. It's a stupid way to learn. A learning curve is much steeper if you learn from the failures and successes of others, too. At the end of the book, I present a few links to the forums I recommend for this purpose. You'll receive the best advice by being specific about your needs and circumstances. Crappy, generic questions ("How to lose weight?") leads to crappy, generic answers ("Quickly!").

7. Find a mentor or an accountability partner online. There are a lot of free weight- loss/fitness forums where people just like you and me share support and experiences. I recommend the same communities which I pointed out as good sources for seeking advice. People there not only know what they are talking about, they are active and caring, too.

My Story

Warning! This chapter is highly redundant with the rest of this book. Many (but not all) pieces of my story were included in some chapters above.

My first real action toward losing weight was a daily portion of pushups. I can't pinpoint the exact time when I started doing this exercise, because I've been doing it (with many breaks) for half my life.

I started doing them for the first time in high school, with this thought: "I'll check how many I can do, and I'll do a little more every week." I started with 40.

I dropped it when I was doing about 120 consecutive pushups.

I started again.

I didn't do them for almost the entire time I was studying at the University.

I started again during my first year of full-time work.

Again, I dropped it.

And about 5.5 years ago, I started it once again and I continue to the present day.

I got up to 130 pushups and changed the strategy, because it was very time-consuming. To start with, I put my feet higher (usually on a bed); later I invited my kids to sit on my back.

And guess what? I didn't lose a single pound.

When I was 16 years old, I injured my spine jumping into a swimming pool. It was nothing serious, but when I got fatter, my spine began to hurt. The pain was annoying, coming back again and again in the least expected moments. One time, the pain almost paralyzed me, so I went to a doctor. She gave me powerful pain killers and said I should work on my belly muscles. I liked the idea of sexy abs instead of a bulging gut, so about 2-2.5 years ago, I started to exercise, working on my belly muscles, 5 minutes a day and ended up exercising 15 minutes a day.

Two things happened then. First - I discovered I actually do have time to work out. To tell the truth, I created my time for workouts. I set an alarm clock 15 minutes earlier. I had already been waking up really early - about 5 am - and 15 minutes didn't make much difference.

Second - I started to gain weight. Very slowly, but steadily. My dark secret is that I have a sweet tooth. I could easily eat two pounds of cake in one afternoon.

There are lessons here, but right now, I'm telling my story, not preaching ;)

I started to pay some attention to what I eat. Five years ago, I used to eat four double sandwiches of white bread at work. I also ate breakfast and a late lunch at home. And a doughnut about every 2-3 days.

And cakes every time there was an occasion to eat one. And some sweets in the evenings. I cut down on white bread, then I replaced it with a dark bread. That was as far as my diet went. ;)

At the beginning of April 2012, I was 163 lbs. It was my peak point. I was even fatter than on my fat photo - I never used to take half-naked pictures of myself, so the last one I have is from a vacation in 2011. As my spine was in no better shape than a year ago, and pain killers prescribed by a doctor were running out, I made the decision to lose weight.

I faced reality. My exercises alone didn't bring me the desired results. And I had no time to exercise more. I needed to change my strategy. I focused on the second element of a weight loss program - the diet. The first thing I did was cut back my consumption of carbs. I gave up 25% of the bread I used to eat. I introduced more vegetables into my eating schedule. I tried to replace sweets with veggies. What a fight it was! Giving up sweets was a constant struggle, not a one-time battle. And it still is. Thanks to those dietary choices, I got some results. In August 2012, I weighed 154 lbs. Nine pounds in 4.5 months - not the most impressive story you've heard about losing weight, is it?

At the end of August, I read a book, which made me take massive action in order to change my life. I set some goals for the first time since ... I don't know exactly, maybe 1999 when I decided on my university studies? One of those goals was my specific weight at the end of the year. I wanted to be 144 lbs.

I didn't introduce many changes this time. I was just more restrictive in my diet. I cut back sweets almost entirely. I started to eat raw carrots as a snack. I tried to compound small activities to add into calories burning - take a walk instead of driving a car, take stairs instead of an elevator, and so on. At the beginning of December 2012, I reached 145 lbs. and hit a plateau. I hadn't achieve my goal, but I was close.

In January 2013, I introduced one new element into my weight-loss program. I started a diet log. It was not rocket science - I simply wrote down everything I ate and drank which contained any calories. I didn't change my diet. I didn't change my work-out regime. I just kept my mind focused on a task by writing down all I ate.

With that, the plateau had been overcome.

On the 12th of January, I reached 144 lbs. By the 9th of March 2013, I was 138 lbs. I lost what I wanted to lose - 15% of my body weight. Since that date, my goal has been to maintain my weight between 138 and 144 lbs. I can proudly state that I haven't even exceeded 141 lbs. since then.

In Conclusion

I've already said what I had to say. Now, it's up to you to take my advice and use it in the way best suited to your temperament, schedule and lifestyle. Your neighbor next door did it. You can do it, too. Go for it! I wish you many pounds lost.

Free Gift for You

Thanks for reading all the way to the end. If you made it this far, you must have liked it!

I really appreciate having people all over the world take interest in the thoughts, ideas, research, and words that I share in my books. I appreciate it so much that I invite you to visit: www.michalzone.com, where you can register to receive all of my future releases absolutely free.

You won't receive any annoying emails or product offers or anything distasteful by being subscribed to my mailing list. This is purely an invite to receive my future book releases for free as a way of saying thanks to you for taking a sincere interest in my work.

Once again, that's www.michalzone.com

A Favor Please

I used to actively discourage my readers from giving me a review immediately after they read my book. I asked you for a review only once you began seeing results. This approach was against common sense and standard practice. Reviews are crucial for a book's visibility on Amazon. And my approach severely hindered me from getting my message out to people just like you, who stand to benefit from it.

I was convinced about that when "Master Your Time in 10 Minutes a Day" became a best-seller. Essentially, I've gotten a number of reviews in a short amount of time, but most of those reviews were the 'plastic' ones we all dislike on Amazon: "Great book! Great content! Great reading! Great entertainment!" Such reviews simply don't carry much weight; anybody could leave a review like that without even reading the book.

In the end, it didn't matter, and my book skyrocketed up the best-seller ranks, anyway. More people than ever have had the chance to get my book in their hands. I'm grateful for this, because more people have received the means to take control over their time and their destiny.

I want to ask a favor of you. If you have found value in this book, please take a moment and share your opinion with the world. Just let me know what you learned and how it affected you in a positive way. Your reviews help me to positively change the lives of others. Thank you!

Recommended Resources for Weight Loss

I'm an outsider. I stumbled and grappled alone to understand what works and what doesn't. I was curious what people gathered in weight loss/fitness forums have to say about my transition – what would be their advice? I did some research while writing this book. I posted a quite detailed description of where I was two years ago, and asked them what to do in my circumstances:

I'm 163 lbs., being 5'5" height. It's about 8 lbs. over BMI's normal weight boundary.

I'm out of shape, because I have little to no time for exercise. I have a sedentary job. I commute about 4 hours a day. Playing with my 3 kids is the most exercise I get.

I didn't pay attention to my diet in the past - my bulging gut is proof of that. What is good - I don't eat fast food, my wife cooks for the whole family. What's bad - I love sweets.

I don't want to be fit overnight. I want to lose weight (about 20 lbs.), be fit and stay that way.

Please advise me what would you recommend and especially what does it mean for me in the terms of daily time investment.

Forums:

If you are looking for an online consultation, I recommend you do the same - give many details, so you'll get a high quality response.

I did it in 6 different online communities. Once, I was totally ignored. Once, I had been given just generic advice. If you want to connect with people who have "been there, done that," find below two forums I recommend:

http://www.fitday.com/fitness/forums/exercise/9 672-how-exercise-very-limited-time.html - great feedback, great advice. One guy even recommended the very exercise I've been doing - pushups. I highly recommend this forum.

http://www.weightlossresources.co.uk - it's a paid service with a free trial. The feedback I got there was a very high quality. They advised me exactly what I did right - a diet log, HIIT training and some mindset tips. Everything that I needed to lose weight. And they did it within 24 hours of the free trial. If you are comfortable with £9,95 monthly fee, go for it!

More Reading:

The Slight Edge by Jeff Olson
The Compound Effect by Darren Hardy
Successful Weight Loss Among Obese U.S. Adults - American Journal of Preventive Medicine

About the Author

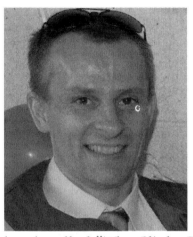

I'm Michal Stawicki and I live in Poland, Europe. I've been married for over 14 years and am the father of two boys and one girl. I work full time in the IT industry, and recently, I've become an author. My passions are transparency, integrity and progress.

In August 2012, I read a book called "The Slight Edge" by Jeff Olson. It took me a whole month to start implementing ideas from this book. That led me to reading numerous other books on personal development, some effective, some not so much. I took a look at myself and decided this was one person who could surely use some development.

In November of 2012, I created my personal mission statement; I consider it the real starting point of my progress. Over several months time, I applied several self-help concepts and started building inspiring results: I lost some weight, greatly increased my savings, built new skills and got rid of bad habits while developing better ones.

I'm very pragmatic, a "down to earth" person. I favor utilitarian, bottom-line results over pure artistry. Despite the ridiculous language, however, I found there is value in the "hokey-pokey visualization" stuff and I now see it as my mission to share what I have learned.

My books are not abstract. I avoid going mystical as much as possible. I don't believe that pure theory is what we need in order to change our lives; the Internet age has proven this quite clearly. What you will find in my books are:

- detailed techniques and methods describing how you can improve your skills and drive results in specific areas of your life
- real life examples
- personal stories

So, whether you are completely new to personal development or have been crazy about the Law of Attraction for years, if you are looking for concrete strategies, you will find them in my books. My writing shows that I am a relatable, ordinary guy and not some ivory tower guru.

Made in the USA
Middletown, DE
22 December 2018